HEALTHWISE

Dorothy Baldwin

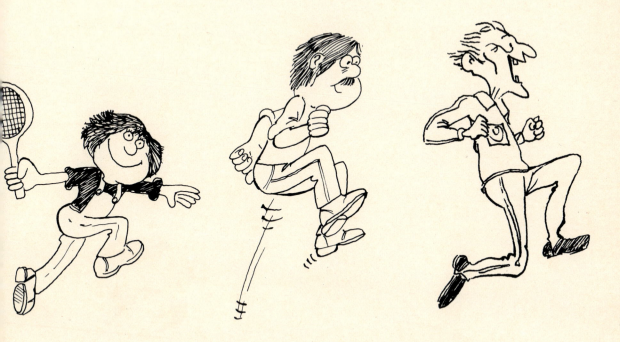

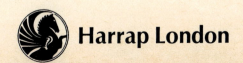
Harrap London

613
833

Acknowledgements

Photographs

Page 4, The Spastics Society; page 5,
National Benevolent Fund for the Aged;
pages 9 and 15, Crown Copyright,
reproduced with the permission of the
Controller of Her Majesty's Stationery
Office; page 17 Tony Othen; page 23,
Department of Medical Illustration,
Institute of Dermatology, London; page 25,
Project Icarus; pages 29, 32, and 33,
Health Education Council; page 30,
Midwives Chronicle; page 31, Camera
Press; page 35, Silhouette Eyewear; page
36, Kangol Helmets Ltd.

This edition first published in Great Britain 1979
by George G. Harrap & Co. Ltd
184 High Holborn, London WC1V 7AX

© George G. Harrap & Co. Ltd, 1979

ISBN 0 245 53336 2

Typeset by Trident Graphics Limited, Reigate

Produced for the publishers by
Linda Rogers Associates
Design: Victor Hazeldine, Peter Sims
Illustrations: Tony Morris, Toni Goffe

Printed and made in Great Britain by
David Green Printers (Limited)
Kettering, Northants

CONTENTS

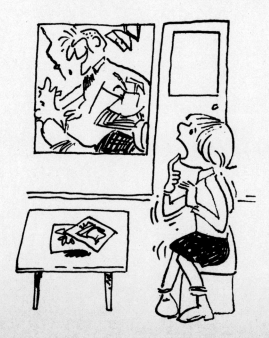

GETTING IT TOGETHER

My name's Sam and I've been going steady with Julie now for quite a time. Julie's great. She must be one of the kindest people ever born. Sometimes she's so soft I feel jealous. She gives too much of her time to other people.

Now, me. I'm the opposite. I'm really quite a selfish person and I wanted Julie to spend more time with me. Especially I wanted her to spend Saturday evenings with me. But she wouldn't. She was off doing voluntary work and though she's kind, like I said, she can be stubborn too. But then so can I. Stubborn as a mule, my Dad used to call me.

Right, I thought, when she had refused to see me for the third Saturday running. I've got to find some way around this little problem. I've got to get it together somehow.

Nobody turns down Sam for long, I promised myself.

This voluntary work Julie does on Saturday nights is to do with a club for the physically handicapped. She goes along, with some friends of hers, to help out, lend a hand, that sort of thing. And she does this, believe it or not, on Saturday evenings!

So I reckoned 'if you can't beat them, join them'. The next week I trailed along behind Julie. As we went into the hall a terrific atmosphere hit us. There were kids in wheel-chairs whizzing around the ping-pong tables playing like mad. There were older ones throwing darts and having the time of their lives. Others were listening to records, playing cards, laughing, talking – even in sign language! The hall was just jumping with life and zest.

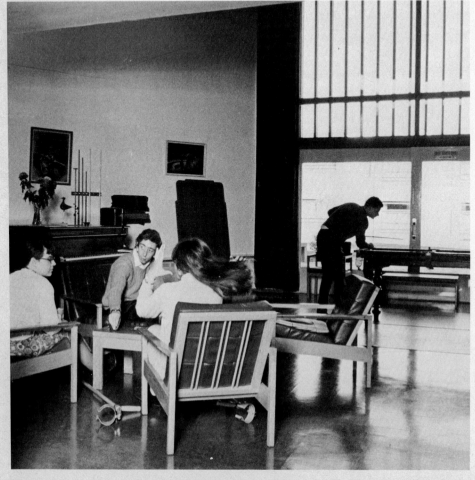

But then a peculiar thing happened to me. In spite of all that happiness I began to feel bad. No, it wasn't jealousy because Julie was so popular. In fact, it had nothing to do with Julie. It was to do with me. I didn't want to be there. I wanted out just as fast as I could.

I couldn't take all those people. There were twisted legs hanging from wheelchairs. There were people not able to see properly, or hear, or talk. There was more damage in that hall than I could bear to think about. And all of these people had great smiles of enjoyment plastered over their faces. I felt very violent and very angry. And I didn't understand why I felt like that.

There was no question about it. I couldn't cope with my own feelings let alone go and play with those kids. I stood around like a spare part waiting for the evening to be over. I didn't want any part of Julie's thing and I wanted her out of it fast.

We had quite a row about it on the way home. I lost, which made me madder than I was before. Julie sat there, all calm and friendly, but refusing to budge. It's difficult to win a row with someone who is so *reasonable*, for heaven's sake.

I had a week to cool off and sort myself out. But it didn't help because I didn't understand my own feelings. Then on the Friday, in our local rag, I saw an ad. asking for volunteers to drive old people out into the country and so on. They wanted volunteers for *Sundays*. This was my chance to get around Julie.

So last Sunday at 3 in the afternoon, Julie and I rang the doorbell of a Mrs. Briggs. She was a trembly old thing and so wobbly on her pins that she was afraid to go out alone — in case she fell over. Julie helped her to put on her hat, one of those crazy jobs with cherries and things bobbing from it. Then off the three of us went in my car.

I couldn't help being touched. Old Mrs. Briggs really got excited by the countryside. She kept calling out the names of flowers and trees as we went along. We stopped just off the road and I cut her a big bunch of ferns. Then we took her back to Julie's house for tea.

Sandra, Julie's kid sister, joined us. She's

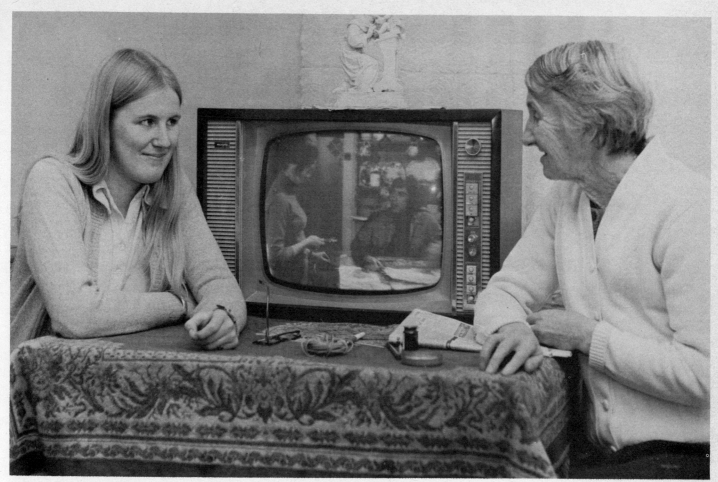

quite a big mouth though she's only sixteen. She told Mrs. Briggs how I felt about helping with damaged kids, and wanting Saturday nights free, and all. I could have killed her.

Mrs. Briggs didn't bat an eyelid. 'Everybody to their liking,' she said, 'why don't you go to this club, Sandra? Let your sister and this nice young man take care of us old things for a change.'

Both Sandra and Julie agreed. Suddenly everything was so simple. I had got it together, hadn't I?

Or had I? Honestly? There's this thought which keeps bugging me, which I don't understand but I know is important.

What I need to know is why I feel so bad when I'm with handicapped people. I just need someone to explain it clearly to me. I'm perfectly happy with the old ladies and gents we take out. But I can't bear to be with young people who are damaged. Why?

Voluntary work is a vital part of community life. Thousands of people spend some time each week helping others. Voluntary work is a two-way business. Both the helper and the helped get satisfaction, pleasure and a sense of belonging and importance in the community. Helping people isn't as simple

as it may appear. It requires time, patience, effort, cheerfulness, reliability and an understanding of other people's needs. Start in a small way, doing something simple such as flag-selling. Then go on to working with people. You can best learn about people's needs by listening carefully to what they tell you.

1. Which age group are you most at ease with; the young, the elderly, your own age?
2. How much time can you spare each week? You *must* turn up regularly.
3. Do you prefer doing something active like cleaning, carpentery, sports?
4. If you are shy, can you find someone to go with you?
5. Are you better at money-raising; raffles, jumbles, sponsored walks, etc.?
6. Do you have the patience to learn the proper way to offer help?
7. Discuss Sam's attitude towards physically handicapped people.

'It's the government's job to look after people, not ours.' What do you think of this statement? What reply would you make?

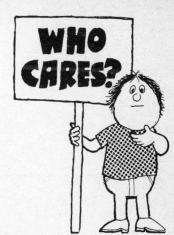

ORGANISED HELP
The Young Volunteer Force and Task Force help young people to find suitable voluntary work. Other well known organisations include the Invalid Children's Aid Association, War on Want, Oxfam, Save the Children, Dr. Barnardo's Homes, Christian Aid, Age Concern and Help the Aged. Some organisations want you to raise money. Others want you to take an active part in their work. The International Voluntary Service will also give advice if you want to work overseas.

YOUR LETTERS........

('Keep on taking the tablets' is such old-fashioned advice that it's become a sort of bad joke. But this isn't true of your letters. Keep on sending them to us. We love getting all your different opinions on health. Sally.)

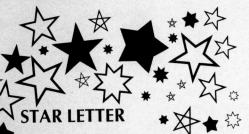

STAR LETTER

Pride comes before a fall
I'm a boy and I don't write letters often but I think this is important. I want to warn anybody who might be going abroad about vaccination. My Dad has a friend living in Kenya, in Nairobi. His son, John, came over to visit us last year and it was my turn to visit him this Christmas.

Everything was fixed. I was so proud of the way I had organised it by myself. I got a fairly cheap flight because I'd booked it so far ahead. My passport cost me £10 and I had to buy some light gear to wear out there. Everything was worked out, down to the last detail, weeks ahead of time.

Then, the night before I was due to leave, an old friend dropped in. He was nearly as excited about my trip as I was. While we were discussing how to take photos of moving animals – I was to go on a safari out there – he suddenly said – 'You've had all your jabs, haven't you?'

A deathly silence followed. My pride rocketed through the floor. I had completely forgotten one of the most important things of all. To get protection against tropical diseases like typhoid and yellow fever. I had to cancel my flight, re-book on a later, more expensive one (I borrowed the extra money from Dad) and get all my jabs as quickly as possible. And that meant my holiday was shortened by a week!

Well, I may not be quite as good at organising as I thought I was – but I'm not stupid about my health. So. Travellers. Beware and make sure you get your jabs. Ask at the travel agency which particular shots you need for whatever foreign country you're going to. Don't get caught as I was!

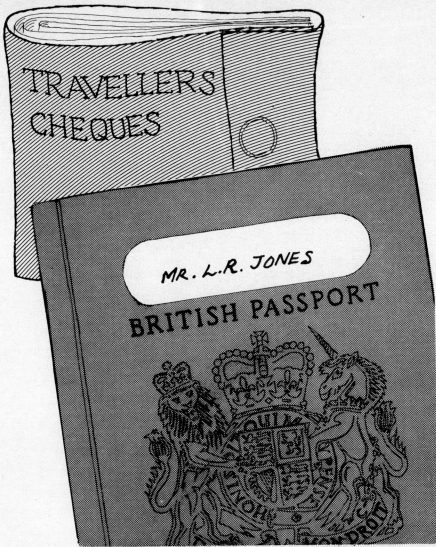

International Health Regulations insist that travellers to, or from, certain countries have valid certificates of vaccination against cholera and yellow fever. If you cannot produce these certificates you may be kept in quarantine for 14 days – at your own expense!

If you visit a country with lower standards of water supply and sewage disposal it is wise to have the typhoid and paratyphoid innoculations as well. (See page 31 for diphtheria and poliomyelitis protection.)

Vaccination requirements change from time to time and from country to country. Get up-to-the-minute information when you book your holiday. Have them done in plenty of time for you to recover from any slight side effects.

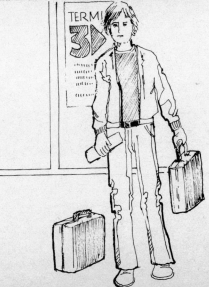

Getting old

I think old age is terrible. Sometimes I watch my Grandad's hands. They are all gnarled and twisted with arthritis and I feel ever so sorry for him. And then, at other times, I get cross with him because it takes him so long to do ordinary simple things. I'm really mixed up. Loving him one day and then not liking him the next day. It makes me feel nervous about getting old myself. I wonder if my grandchildren will think of me the same as I think of my Grandad.

I know a lot of old people who have arthritis. I'm worried in case I get it when I'm old. My Grandad says I won't because of the central heating but I'm not sure he knows what he's talking about. So I asked the P.E. master and he said the best thing was to do exercise and sports. Right through your life, he said. (Not that it stops arthritis – the doctors don't understand enough about it yet.) But exercise keeps your body firm and flexible. Too many people stop taking exercise when they leave school. I have made a firm resolution. Look out for me when I'm fifty, jogging around the park in my old track suit!

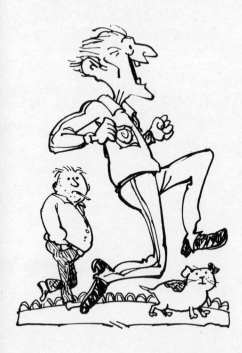

Discuss how you feel about old age. 'The majority of people stop taking exercise once they leave school.' Will you? Find out about yoga and isometrics. Write to the Physical Education Association for information on more unusual sports like canoeing, pony-trekking, skin-diving, mountaineering, etc.

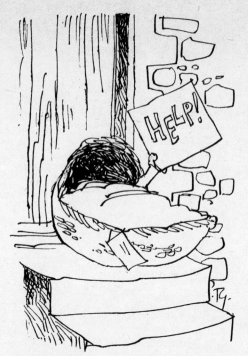

Orphan Annie

I am fed up with hearing about people having babies without being married. Everyone is so sympathetic to the lady, worrying and fussing about her. It makes me sick. I think, 'What about that poor baby? What sort of life is it going to have?'

I had it rough myself as my mother wasn't married. She kept me for a while then put me in a Home. After that I went to foster parents. I couldn't get on with them and had to be sent back to the Home. It wasn't their fault. It was mine. I didn't behave very well. I kept thinking, 'I should be with my real Mum.' Which was daft, 'cause I'd almost forgotten what she looked like.

Well, I'm older now and more sensible. But I still feel very bitter and angry sometimes. I even feel bitter towards my father – whoever he may be! We had a lesson the other day and were told you can get birth control free from the clinic. We were also told that people still go on having unwanted babies. Honestly, it made me mad. When I thought of all those little babies and my own rotten childhood, I wanted to cry.

Please. Let's not go on handing out sympathy to unmarried mothers. It just encourages other people to behave in the same way. My friends think I'm hard and cruel. I think their soppiness adds to the unhappiness of the world. I know what I'm talking about.

Discuss 'Orphan Annie's' experience as a child and the way she feels now. What do you think of her sentence 'It just encourages other people to behave in the same way'?

Ear hole

Four girls pierced their ears a couple of weeks ago. They did it in break-time with a needle. Now three of them have huge sores and can't wear their 'sleepers'. Ear piercing is barbaric. They might as well stick bones through their noses. Fancy making holes in perfectly healthy flesh! I can't understand it.

Whenever the skin is broken open there is *always* a risk of infection. All wounds, cuts, scratches (and deliberately-made holes) should be bathed with an antiseptic lotion to kill off any germs and then covered in plaster to prevent other germs from getting in. As this is not possible in ear-piercing many people suffer from infected lobes.

Catching

My friends and I are very healthy. Last week I got hold of a book on diseases. It was really unpleasant to read. But we couldn't stop ourselves. We went right through the book from beginning to end. And then we began thinking we might have some of those diseases!

I am now certain that teaching young people about illnesses is not good for them. It is easy to imagine you have a secret disease yourself. I think the less you know about such things the better. I wonder if your readers agree with me.

The most important part of 'Healthwise' is to *prevent* illness by understanding more about it. Do you think people are likely to feel frightened if they know more – or less – about certain diseases? *Hypochondria* is unnecessary anxiety over health. It is also imaginary feelings of being unwell. Have you ever had a mild twinge of hypochondria!

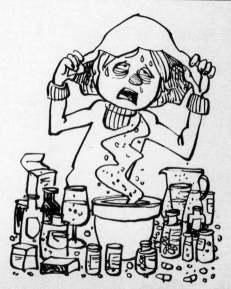

Dreaded dentist

This is a letter from a coward. A real one hundred percent 'jelly baby'. I am terrified of going to the dentist. A lot of people tell me they are frightened. My feelings are much stronger than that. I am really and truly terrified.

I put off going until I can't stand the pain of toothache anymore. Then, while I am sitting in the dentist's waiting room, I hear the shrill whine of the drill being used. Shudders run down me and I clench my hands so tightly they go white. Once I actually dug my nails right into my palm. All this before I even see him.

At last I am sitting in the chair and he is probing in my mouth with that pick thing. I start to wriggle and squirm before he has hurt me. I am such a coward. At last, I can stand it no more. Whether he is hurting me or not, I begin to cry. I can feel the tears rising up, no matter how hard I try to keep them back. It is most humiliating to cry in the dentist.

I told my Mum I couldn't bear going to the dentist anymore. I said I was going to have all my teeth taken out and have false ones. Then I'd have no more trouble.

A curious and embarrassing thing happened. She – my Mum, I mean – she began to cry; great huge sobs. I didn't know what to do. Then she took out her false teeth and made me look at her face without them. It really did look awful; drawn in and old and sort of withered. I hadn't realised that it's the roots of your teeth which keep your jaws nice and firm.

She didn't say anything to me. She didn't have to! She just sat there, with tears running down into the wrinkles and puckers round her gummy mouth. She's a wonderful Mum. Showing me how awful she looked and how bad she felt about losing her teeth. That must have taken some courage. Now I'll have to go to the dentist again, won't I? You see, I can't be less brave than my Mum. I owe her that. But, oh dear, I get the shakes at the very thought of the 'dreaded dentist'.

By the age of forty 50% of people in the Western world have no teeth left. They wear dentures. What is your opinion of the way this mother *without saying anything* gave her daughter the courage to continue having dental treatment? Treatment is free for the under 21's, for pregnant women and those with a baby under a year old.

The kissing disease

I have got glandular fever and a wonderful doctor. First I had a high fever, a splitting headache and sore throat. That lasted for a week and was called the acute stage. Then, my temperature dropped and I got better though I felt tired and had no energy for ages after. I was off school with it for three months and missed my exams.

My doctor said it is a funny disease because some people get it as badly as I did. Others are hardly unwell at all. Unfair! He says the only way they can tell if you have glandular fever or not is by taking some of your blood. It shows in the white blood cells. I must admit I didn't enjoy having my blood taken.

Anyway, there isn't much you can do except wait to recover. My friend Suzy came to visit me. She'd had it mildly and called it the kissing disease. I couldn't believe my ears! We had quite a little argument about it. Finally, I plucked up courage and asked my smashing doctor. I could feel myself blushing all over. Kissing disease indeed!

He laughed. He said it is a common disease in young adults and maybe that was how it got its nick-name. He said he'd had it long before he knew about kissing. But he gave me such a cheeky grin I didn't know if he was teasing or not. Now Suzy tells me I've got a crush on him. Well, what with one thing and another, I must admit it is a funny disease.

Doctors are still not sure what causes glandular fever. The popular theory is that it is caused by a virus – the smallest germs. Some young people have quite severe attacks while others may not even notice they have anything wrong. It is not a serious disease but it can cause great inconvenience – missing exams, job opportunities and so on.

Scared

I had to wait nine months before having my tonsils out. They were the longest months of my life. Being a boy you're not supposed to be scared of anything. So I didn't dare to tell how I felt about having 'gas'. Scared silly, that's how I was. And for nine long months too.

Now it's over I don't mind talking about it. I would like to tell anyone in my position i.e. waiting for an operation, that there is nothing to be afraid of. You see, I was scared of being put to sleep, of being given the wrong gas or something like that. I was scared I would never wake up again.

In fact what happened was simple. The nurse gave me an injection which made me feel calm and happy and sleepy. After a while I was put on a trolley. I was wheeled along corridors and into a little room near the operating theatre. The man who gives the gas is called an anaesthetist. He was dressed in green and was a hearty sort of bloke. He gave me another injection. No, he didn't tell me to count from a hundred downwards. He told me to count up to ten. I got as far as three and floated off into a weird dream.

That's all there was to it. I woke up in my bed again, a bit sick and with a horrible sore throat. But the relief was fantastic. No more worry. I would have given three loud cheers if my throat hadn't been so sore!

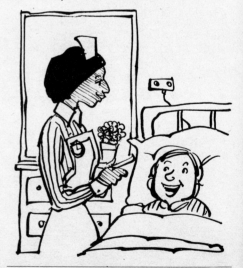

Anaesthetics are drugs used to 'deaden' nerves so the patient feels no pain. A *general* anaesthetic is used in large operations and puts the patient into a deep sleep. A *spinal* anaesthetic deadens the nerves below the place where it is injected. It is sometimes used in childbirth – the mother is wide awake but feels no pain. A *local* anaesthetic is injected into a small area e.g. one side of the mouth. It is often used by dentists.

Blood wanted

Some years ago I had a bad accident. I fell over as I was carrying the milk bottles. They smashed on the concrete ground outside our flat. A huge piece of glass went right into my wrist and stuck out, all jagged. Blood poured everywhere. The funny thing was, I didn't feel any pain. I'm told I fainted away ever so gracefully.

In the hospital I had to be given two bottles of blood. To make up what I'd lost. As I lay there, watching some other human's blood dripping into me, I tried to imagine who that person was. I thought whoever it was, he or she was good and kind and helpful. I mean, there was I getting this blood, thanks to their generosity.

The point is this. I think everyone should give blood as soon as they are old enough. I've found out the details for your readers. You have to be over 18, in normal health and not suffering from certain diseases. When you get to the Blood Doning Centre they take a pin-prick of blood to test it. Then you lie down and give about two cupfuls through a needle in your arm. The donor rests for a while and is given tea or coffee and biscuits. The whole business only lasts about half an hour and then you go back to work. Your body soon makes up the blood you have given.

Go on. Be generous. Give blood. You can afford it.

Becoming a blood donor at 18 is an extremely valuable community service. The blood is kept in special 'blood banks' in hospitals. Can you imagine what might happen if healthy people stopped giving their blood? Another important donor scheme is for kidney transplants. The donors carry a card giving permission for their kidneys to be removed and transplanted into a kidney patient – in the case of their sudden death.

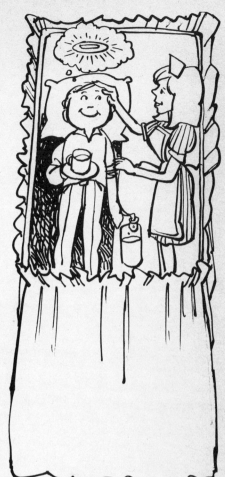

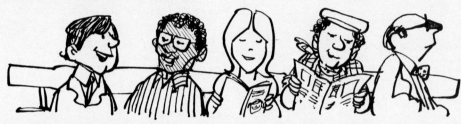

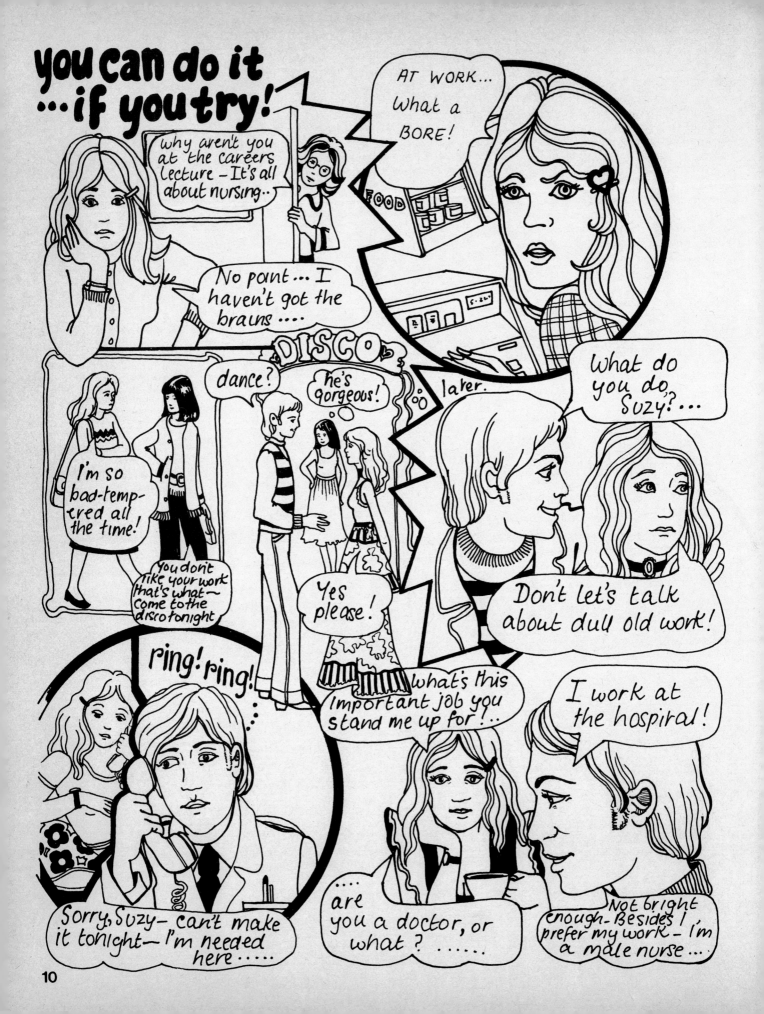

you can do it ...if you try!

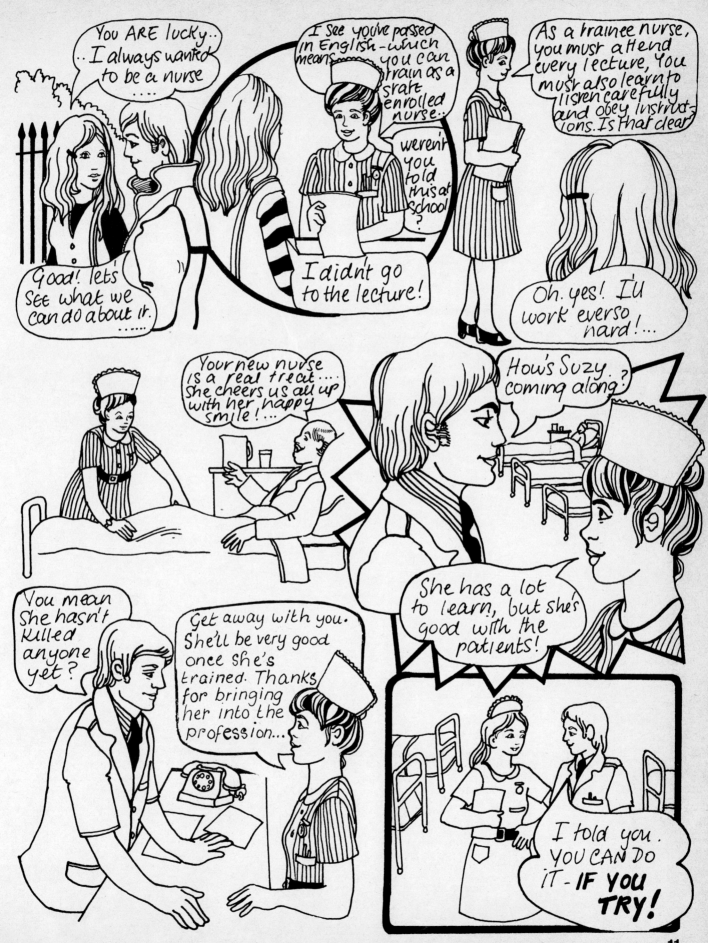

You can do it if you try

is a fairy-tale story. It is quite rare to get a second chance as Suzy did. But it is true that many young people miss the opportunities of doing work they would enjoy. One reason is the urge to rush out and earn your own money as soon as possible. Another reason, as in Suzy's story, is lack of confidence. Always attend careers talks and your career interviews. You never can tell what you can do till you try.

Hospitals are friendly, busy places to work in. There is usually quite a bit of discipline as it is vital each person does the work properly. In spite of this people choose to work in hospitals because of the cheerful helpful atmosphere. There are many jobs which do not need special exam qualifications. Ambulance drivers, porters, photographers, office staff, technicians and maintenance workers do need training. Ward orderlies, canteen workers, kitchen cleaners and domestic staff can learn the job as they gain experience.

FIGUREWISE

At this moment the lunch you ate yesterday is being turned into energy, new cells, body juices, tiny parts of eyelashes, skin, muscle, teeth, etc. We are rather like huge chemical factories. We take in food to produce healthy and active human bodies and minds. What did you eat for lunch yesterday?

There's no prize for guessing what happens if we don't take in the right amounts of the right foods! Some part of us – maybe many years from now – will stop working properly. We suffer from a food deficiency disease. This is why it is important you learn the 'Facts on Food'. And why you must eat a *balanced* diet – plenty of different *kinds* of food. For your health's sake.

Another important point to remember is that you will *look* more attractive. Your skin will be clearer, your hair glossier, your eyes more sparkling. You will have more energy, more vivacity, more fun out of being alive.

NOT TOO LITTLE (Anorexia Nervosa)
This is a sad and rare disorder found in a few teenage girls and young women. It is an extreme dislike of eating and is caused by some deep mental disturbance. As the patient eats less and less her body weight drops, her muscles wither, her skin dries and ages, her hair falls out. Her periods stop and so does her development. However she *insists* she is feeling fine and she is eating properly.

If she is determined not to eat at all, she will starve herself to death. An anorexic person needs immediate psychiatric help. It is a very difficult disorder to treat as the person often does not want to be helped.

NOT TOO MUCH (Obesity)
This is a sad but fairly common disorder. It is very easily put right though it does need an enormous amount of self-discipline. Don't blame your glands; blame your eating habits. You are simply taking in more food than your body can use. The extra food is stored as fat. Fat people tend to have a slower rate of 'burning up' food than slim people. Remember this, especially when you are feeling hungry. *You need to eat less.*

Don't go on crash diets – they don't work. Stop eating fried foods (chips) and really cut down your intake of starches and sugars. But do it *slowly*, eating a little less each *week*. Obesity is associated with heart disease and diabetes in later life. It is important you lose extra weight now. But don't be cruel to yourself. *Take slimming slowly.*

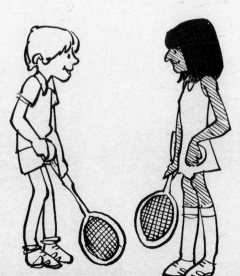

BUT JUST RIGHT (Who's perfect?)
Between these two extremes people come in all shapes, sizes and weights! There is no such thing as a perfect figure. Film stars often have bits taken off and sewn on to other places! Don't waste time longing for a perfect figure. Be happy with what you've got. Exercise it every day. Feed it a balanced diet. Keep it clean and fresh. Then relax and enjoy it.

Love me – love my figure 'faults and all' is the best attitude.

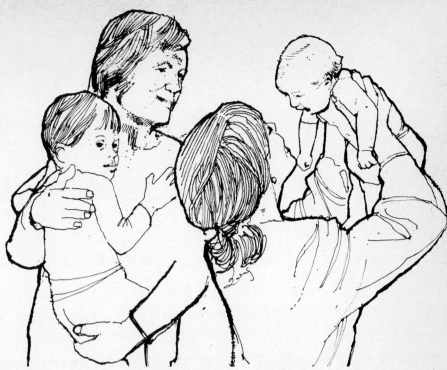

ALL YOU NEED IS LOVE

Like many sayings this is not quite the whole truth. Babies and small children need more than love. They need *understanding*. It is now known that the first years of life are extremely important for the healthy development of the mind. A very 'bad' experience in early life may cause mental illness later on. From birth a baby needs to feel he belongs to his mother and his family. He needs to learn trust and love. He needs cuddles and company. He needs to feel he is a 'good' person living in a 'safe' world. This will help him to grow into a confident and secure adult. Understanding a child's emotional needs is a vital part of being a good parent. Society is beginning to help parents of the future by encouraging Child Development to be taught in schools and colleges.

MENTAL HANDICAP

Mental illness is *not* the same as mental handicap. You can recover from a mental illness; you cannot recover from a mental handicap. Once the brain is severely damaged it cannot mend itself. About 4 in every 1,000 babies are born with brain damage.

For reasons not yet known the brain cells of these babies do not develop properly before birth. Brain damage can also be caused by severe head injuries – often from road accidents. It also happens when the heart stops beating. When blood stops being pumped to the brain the cells begin to be destroyed after about 3 minutes. People with brain damage are not mentally ill – they are mentally handicapped.

Mental Illness isolates

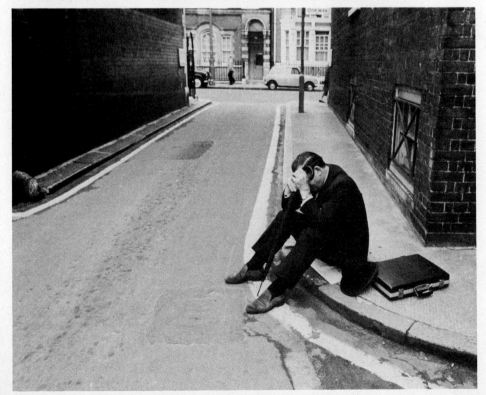

Points for discussion and projects.

1. The difference between mental illness and mental handicap.
2. Schools and homes for the mentally-handicapped child.
3. The teaching of Child Development in colleges and schools.
4. Baby-Battering or Non-Accidental Injuries.
5. Children's Homes, Fostering and Adoption.
6. State Nurseries and Baby Minders.
7. The Working Mother and the One Parent Family.
8. Playgroups and Adventure Playgrounds.
9. The National Society for the Prevention of Cruelty to Children (NSPCC).
10. The Invalid Children's Aid Association (ICAA).
11. The National Association for Mental Health (MIND).

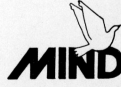

MIND

Mental Health needs good neighbours

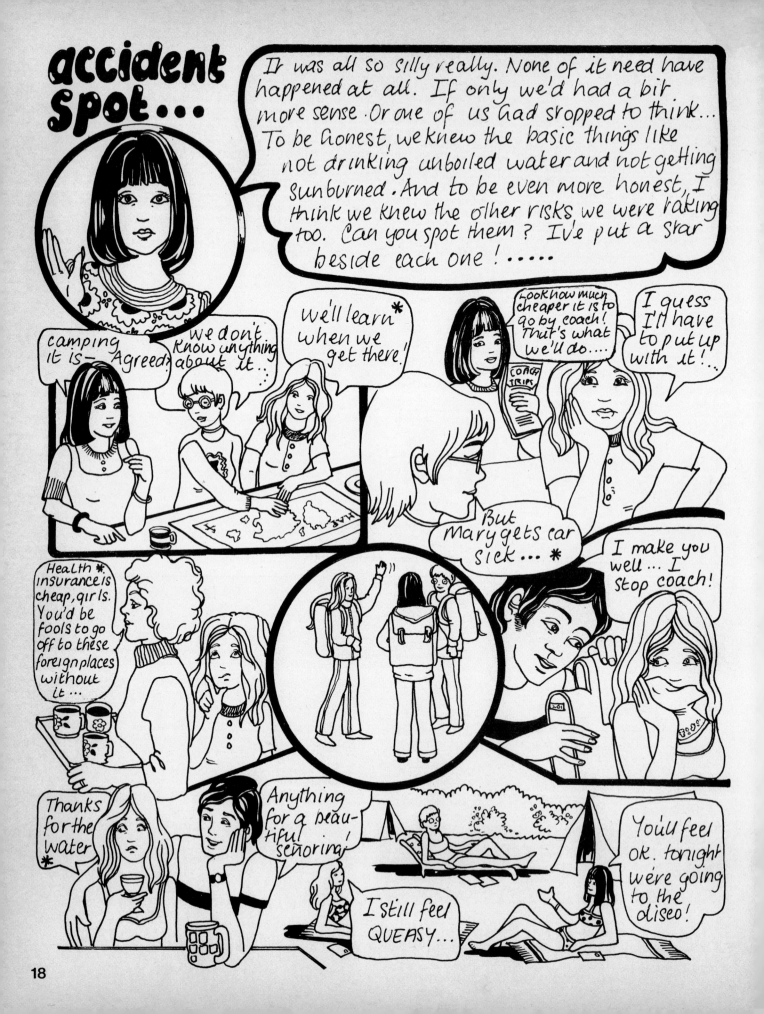

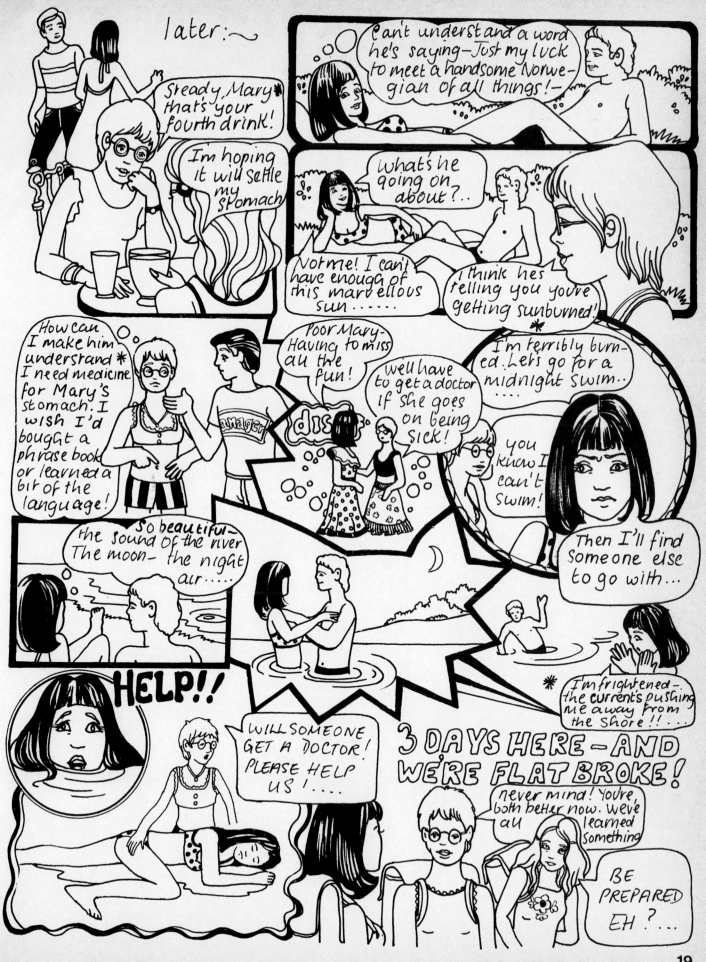

ACCIDENT SPOT

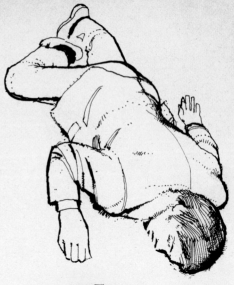

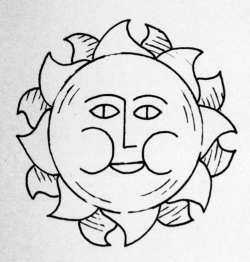

FOR HOLIDAYS IN THE SUN

1. Take your first aid kit. Add to it travel-sick pills, sun creams and oils, calamine lotion, insect repellant ointment and anti-'runs'–diarrhoea tablets.
2. Don't stay in the sun too long. Get acclimatised (used to the different climate) slowly.
3. Drink plenty of fluids. 2 litres a day for basic needs and 1 litre for every 10 deg.C increase in the temperature. Go easy on alcoholic drinks.
4. Drinking water must be boiled or buy bottled mineral water.
5. Peel fresh fruit. Meat and fish should be thoroughly cooked. Avoid ice lollies.
6. Add plenty of salt to your food to put back what you lose in sweating.
7. Wear loose cotton-mix clothes. Never wear pure nylon.
8. Learn a few of the essential words and take a phrase book with you.
9. Always take out private health insurance. This covers you against illness and accident for a very low fee. E.E.C. countries now have a 'swop' arrangement with the U.K. for free treatment but there are many conditions which you must fulfil first.
10. Know what to do in an emergency.

WHAT TO DO IN AN EMERGENCY

1. When breathing has stopped. Act immediately because of the certain risk of brain damage. Check there is nothing blocking the air passages and start artificial respiration. Do not stop till the person begins breathing or till help arrives.

2. Breathing but unconscious. Turn the person to the recovery position, head tipped slightly downwards. Cover with a light blanket or coat. Send for an ambulance. (Never turn an unconscious person on his back. If he vomits, as in drug overdose, he will inhale it and suffocate.)

3. Heavy bleeding. Make a pad from some clean cloth and press this down firmly on the wound. Keep on pressing down. Get the person to hospital for the wound to be stitched.

4. Broken bones. Keep the fractured part absolutely still. If it is an open fracture cover the wound with a clean cloth. Call an ambulance.

5. Serious burns. Hold the burned area under the cold water tap. Continue cooling for ten minutes. Get the person to hospital as soon as possible. Give sips of water to *conscious* patient. (The *only* time you can give something to drink in *any* serious emergency is when someone is badly burned.)

For further study read *New Safety and First Aid* by Gardner & Roylance, Pan. You should however enrol for a proper first aid course so that you always know exactly what to do in an emergency. You will also be taught how to treat minor injuries.

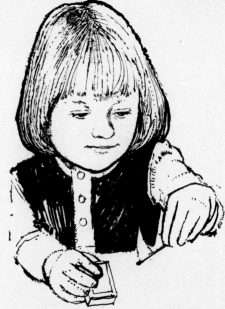

SAFETY AT HOME

Home, sweet home, is the most dangerous place for accidents. Babies, small children and old people are most at risk. Why do you think this is so? Write to RoSPA for information on safety in the home.

SAFETY ON THE ROAD

Do you think it is right we should have to wear seat-belts? Find out the penalty for not wearing a crash-helmet when riding a motor-bike. How would you set about teaching a small child road safety? It is an offence to drive with more than 80 milligrams of alcohol in 100 millilitres of blood. Why is it an offence?

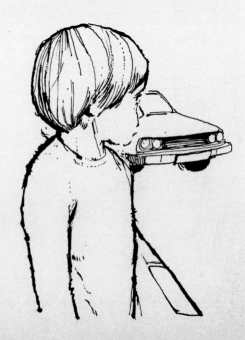

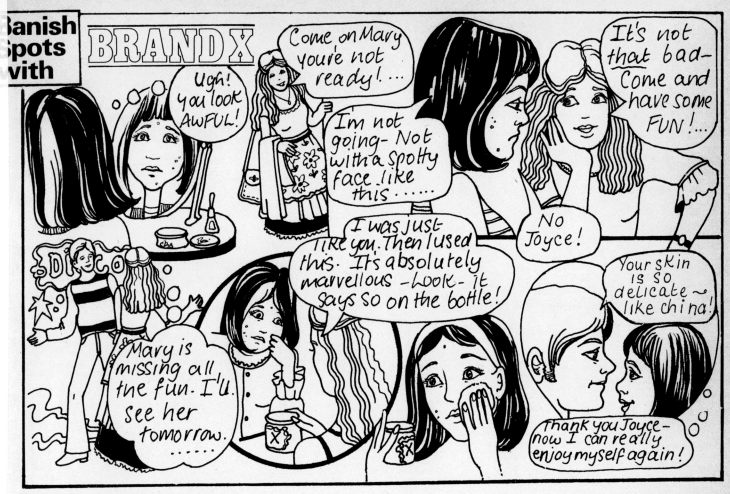

In advertisements like this it is always a *girl* who is shown to be the spotty one. In real life boys get acne just as often and just as badly as girls.

Infections of the skin

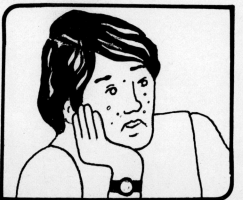

The most usual place for acne is the forehead, the sides of the nose, the jaw line and the chin. It can also spread to the neck, shoulders, chest and back. Most people have at least one attack during the mid or late teens. Acne is caused by the change of hormones during adolescence and by the sweat and oil glands working overtime. (Other reasons include eating too much fried food and chocolate, not eating enough fresh fruit and vegetables, lack of fresh air and exercise. But these things will *not* cause acne by themselves.)

ACNE STARTS WITH SPOTS

Spots can be whiteheads, pimples, blackheads or angry-looking lumps under the skin. If you are unlucky, you may get all of these at the same time.

Spots happen because:

Oil glands in the skin make an oil called sebum. Sebum keeps the hair and skin oiled and smooth. When the oil glands work overtime too much oil is made. *It forms a greasy film on the skin.*

Sweat glands get rid of heat, a little water and tiny amounts of body waste. Some people sweat quite heavily in their teens, especially when they are nervous, embarrassed or excited. *The tiny amounts of body waste mix with the greasy film.*

The top level of the skin is covered with dead cells. *These also mix with the body waste and greasy film.*

During the teens the texture of the skin changes slightly. It becomes a little thicker. (Look at a child's skin to compare.) While it is changing the oil may not be able to get through to the surface. The pores get blocked with dried oil. Waste, dead cells and dirt from the air plug up the opening of the blocked pores. *All this makes a perfect breeding ground for germs.*

STOP THOSE SPOTS

From the beginning of the teens the face should be washed frequently. Start by washing your hands thoroughly. Then, using plenty of warm, soapy suds, really clean the whole of the face and neck area for two minutes. (Don't use a flannel unless you boil it each week – it could be full of germs. Don't use a scented soap – it could irritate the skin.) Rinse thoroughly by splashing on luke-warm water for one minute. Rub briskly with a towel to dry. Or, pat gently if you have a dry, sensitive skin. If you wash away the dead cells, the body waste and the greasy film you could have a clear complexion right through your teens.

THE SPOT PICKER

Careless picking of spots causes acne. The spot picker squeezes a spot, pushing grime from the fingers and face into it. The spot cannot heal as it is full of germs. The spot picker then has a go at another spot. And another. Soon the whole face is infected. The person suffers a nasty attack of acne.

It seems crazy but this is what many people actually do. They infect their own skin! They cause their own acne!

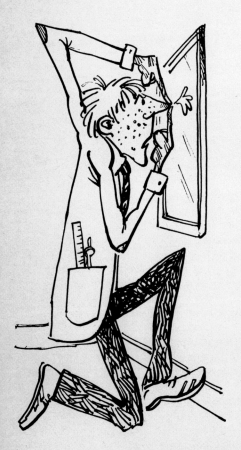

SPOT TREATMENT

1. Wash your face till it is completely clean.
2. Scrub your hands, fingertips and nails.
3. Soak a piece of cotton wool in hot water and press it over the spot. This will soften the skin.
4. *Gently* squeeze the spot out by pressing *gently* on the area around it.
5. Dab a little antiseptic on the open pore. This will help it to close and stop other germs getting in.
6. Only treat one spot at a time.
7. Wash hands again before touching another spot.
8. Never touch spots absent-mindedly.

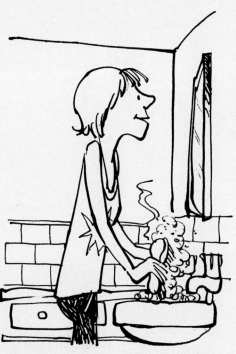

DOES BRAND X IN THE ADVERTISEMENT REALLY WORK?

Yes and no. It depends on your type of skin. Each person's skin has a different chemical balance and what suits one person may be bad for another. And if there were a wonder cure for acne then nobody would have it after the first few days.

Stick to the daily routine of washing and rinsing for at least three months. If your skin is dry wipe on a little cream or lotion. Otherwise leave your skin alone.

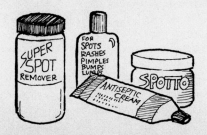

WHAT HAPPENS IF I DO GET ACNE?

If it is *very bad* ask your doctor for help. The ointment you will be given is very powerful. Use it sparingly and for a short time only. If you put on too much – or for too long – it may damage your skin. Never use a friend's ointment. It could be just the wrong thing for your skin.

SWEATING

Sweating is another problem of adolescence. During the early teens new sweat glands begin to work. The most noticeable ones are on the feet, in the groin, under the arms and on the palms of the hands. Fresh sweat doesn't smell. Stale sweat does. Washing all over each day is essential.

Being clean doesn't mean just not getting dirty. Being clean means removing your own sweat, dead cells and body oils by washing them off the skin *every day*. Being clean means changing your underwear each day. Clothes which touch your skin mop up some of your body grime. Being clean means washing your hair regularly. Being clean means having strict personal hygiene before you touch food and after you've used the toilet. Being clean means being safe from skin infections.

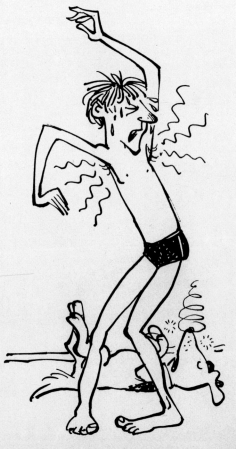

RINGWORM – ANOTHER SKIN INFECTION

Ringworm sounds more horrid than it really is. There are no worms in ringworm. It is a skin infection of *fungus* which spreads out into something like a circle. There are two kinds which infect teenagers, athlete's foot and ringworm of the leg.

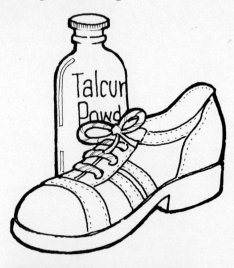

ATHLETE'S FOOT

You can catch this infection whether you are athletic or not! The fungus is picked up when you walk barefoot – especially in public baths and showers. You can also pick it up by borrowing towels or shoes from someone who has the infection.

The first thing you may notice are small cracks between the toes. The cracks open, the skin goes whitish and 'weeps'. Then it peels off leaving raw, red patches which are itchy. Or it may start as small yellow blisters on the soles of the feet. They spread to the heels and make them sore.

Treatment:
Ask the chemist for an ointment to kill off the fungus. If you get another attack ask your doctor for something stronger. Keep your feet cool, dry and clean. Wash them every day and when they get hot after exercise. Dry them carefully especially between the toes. Then dust all over with talcum powder. Socks or tights must be changed every day. It takes a bit of time and patience to get rid of athlete's foot.

RINGWORM OF THE LEG

This type of fungus infection is caught mainly by teenage boys and young men. It is picked up in schools, colleges and clubs where sports clothes and towels are shared. It may also be caught from toilet seats in these places. It is more usual to catch it in the summer months.

It begins high up near the groin on the inside of the leg. The first thing you notice is a small, red, slightly bumpy patch on the skin. This patch grows and spreads down the inside thigh for 5 to 7mm. It looks very nasty but it's not serious.

Treatment:
This may take even longer to clear up as your trousers will rub against the patch and spread the fungus. Wear shorts or swimming trunks whenever it's possible. Get ointment or tablets from your doctor and follow the instructions very carefully.

(Ringworm of the scalp is usually only caught by young children.)

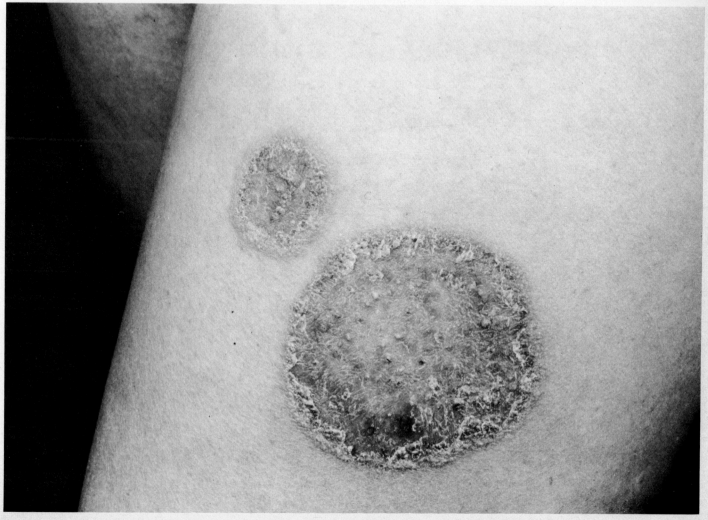

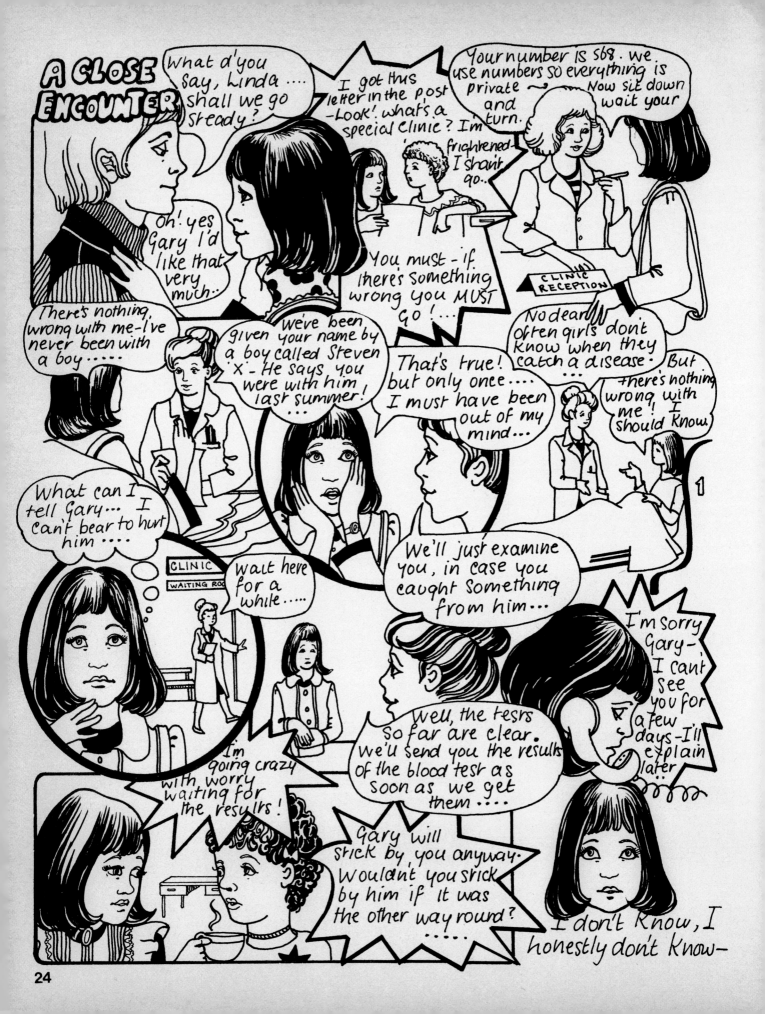

Sexually Transmitted Diseases

THE FACTS

Sex diseases are called sexually-transmitted diseases. (STD for short.) They are passed directly from one person to another.

It is *very rare* to pick them up from towels, toilet seats or door handles.

STD germs die when they are not on the human body.

Almost as many people catch an STD as catch measles.

The number of cases amongst young adults is rising steadily.

Men usually know when they have an STD. They can see the sores – they can feel the pain when passing water.

Women often don't know when they have an STD. If the infection is inside their body, they may have no signs of disease.

An STD will not clear up by itself without special treatment. The longer it is left untreated the worse it will get.

All STD can be cured if they are treated at once. An untreated STD will cause serious health problems later on.

THE SPECIAL CLINICS

These are usually attached to a hospital.

They are for treating any infections of the sex organs.

Anyone can go to a special clinic without an appointment.

The patient is given a number to keep his/her identity a secret.

A doctor examines the patient carefully. If a disease is found the patient is given immediate treatment.

The patient must tell the person from whom he/she has caught the disease. This is vital as he/she may not know about STD.

Both the patient and his/her contact are responsible to the community. They must not spread the disease any further.

The staff at special clinics are gentle and helpful.

Treatment is free. It is paid for by the working members of society.

POINTS TO REMEMBER

Pain in passing water is a sign that something is going wrong. (Pain is not only caused by an STD.)

Discharge is a creamy fluid to keep the woman's vagina healthy and clean. If discharge becomes very heavy or unpleasant smelling, it may also be a warning that something is going wrong.

Only a specially trained person can diagnose (find out) an STD. STD germs are found in the blood and/or the discharge of the patient.

The chart in the summary is *not* for diagnosis; simply for information. If a person has any cause for worry, he/she should go to the clinic at once.

GENERAL HYGIENE OF THE SEX ORGANS

Germs breed rapidly in the area around the sex organs. Strict personal hygiene, washing the area every day, is a *must* for *everyone*. Underclothes should be changed every day. This stops germs which are *not* STD's from causing any skin infections.

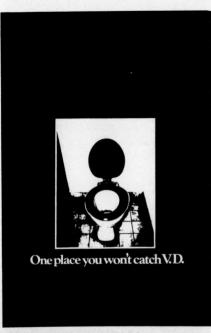

One place you won't catch V.D.

V.D. is a sexually transmitted disease. It can only be caught through direct bodily contact.
If you put yourself at risk, have a check up. It makes sense to make sure.

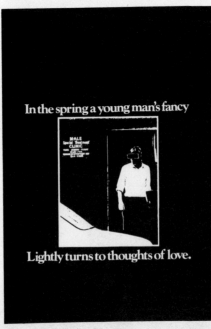

In the spring a young man's fancy

Lightly turns to thoughts of love.

The treatment of V.D. is safe, simple and costs nothing.
If you put yourself at risk, have a check up. It makes sense to make sure.

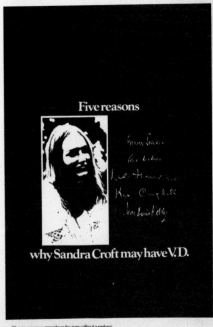

Five reasons

why Sandra Croft may have V.D.

Women can carry gonorrhoea for years without symptoms.
If you put yourself at risk, have a check up. It makes sense to make sure.

sexually transmitted diseases

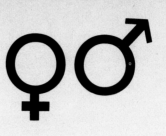

NAME	FIRST SIGNS	TREATMENT	UNTREATED DISEASE
Syphilis (pox)	Men: Painless sore on penis. Women: Painless sore on or inside sex organs.	Blood test followed by course of injections. Check-ups till clear.	Sore disappears. Germs get into blood and taken all over body. In late stage, blindness, insanity, paralysis – death.
Gonorrhoea (clap)	Men: Pain when passing water. Pus from penis. Women: 70% have no signs at all. An increase in discharge, pain.	Discharge or pus tested. Short course of injections or tablets. Check-ups.	Germs travel up into sex organs and breed. Causes scarring of tubes. Both men and women get infertile (unable to have children)
Non-specific urethritis (NSU)	Men: Pain when passing water. Pus and discharge from penis. Women: —	Different methods of treatment.	Disease of joints. Infections of eyes, skin. Other problems.

LESS SERIOUS INFECTIOUS DISEASES

NAME	FIRST SIGNS	TREATMENT	UNTREATED DISEASE
Trichomoniasis vaginalis (TV)	Men: — Women: Pain and itchiness. Discharge very unpleasant.	A course of tablets till check-up is clear.	Continuing pain and nasty discharge from vagina.
Candidiosis (thrush)	Men: Tip of penis sore. Women: Heavy discharge, sore.	2 weeks course of special tablets put inside vagina.	Women can get thrush from illness, taking certain medicines, etc. Thrush is *not* always an STD.
Warts	Small round raised growths on sex organs.	Special lotions from clinic. Strict personal hygiene.	Other germs may get in and cause far more serious trouble.
Herpes	Germs which cause sores like cold sores on sex organs.	Strict personal hygiene.	Other germs can get into the sores.
Lice (crabs)	Like head lice but live in pubic hair. Very itchy.	Shave off all pubic hair. Wash in D.D.T. lotion. Strict personal hygiene.	Lice feed off blood so whole area at risk from other germs.
Scabies	Tiny bugs which burrow under skin and lay eggs there. Itchiness and soreness.	Strong lotions from chemist or clinic. Strict personal hygiene.	Also blood-suckers. Difficult to get rid of as eggs underneath skin. Best to have treated at special clinic.

HOW HEALTHWISE ARE YOU?

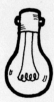

When you study under electric light where should the light fall:
- a) Onto the work you are doing?
- b) Beside you?
- c) In front of you?

When you have a headache do you:
- a) Work out what's caused it then try to avoid doing whatever it was?
- b) Take tablets to stop the pain and carry on?
- c) Lie down and make a fuss of yourself?

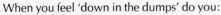

An old man falls down unconscious in the street. Would you:
- a) Turn him to the recovery position?
- b) Ask a passer-by to help?
- c) Feel embarrassed and walk on?

When you feel 'down in the dumps' do you:
- a) Tell yourself it's only a mood and it will pass?
- b) Rush out and buy something to cheer yourself up?
- c) Wallow in self-pity till you feel full of gloom and despair?

Which of these is the best balanced meal when you are eating out:
- a) Hamburger, salad and milk shake?
- b) Fish and chips and tea?
- c) Meat pie, pickled onions and a lager?

Do you visit the dentist:
- a) Every six months?
- b) Only when you have toothache?
- c) Never?

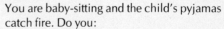

You are baby-sitting and the child's pyjamas catch fire. Do you:
- a) Throw a blanket over him to cut off the oxygen?
- b) Throw water over him to put out the flames?
- c) Rush into the bedroom to see what started the fire?

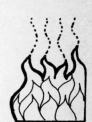

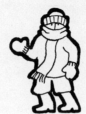

Which will keep you warmest in winter:
- a) Two layers of woollen clothes?
- b) Three layers of cotton and nylon mix clothes?
- c) Four layers of nylon clothes?

If you had a persistent pain would you:
- a) Go to the doctor?
- b) Look up a medical book for signs and symptoms of disease?
- c) Worry in secret that you have some dreadful illness?

If you only had enough water to do one of these things would you:
- a) Wash your body?
- b) Wash your hair?
- c) Wash your underclothes?

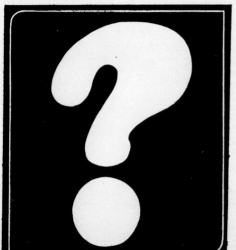

If you answered all a) questions then you have a sound and sensible attitude to health. Furthermore it seems you are prepared to do what is necessary in an emergency as well as what is plain common-sense at other times. You are likely to be a cool, well-balanced person if you continue to use your judgement wisely.

If you answered mainly b) questions then you've quite a bit of common-sense but you're not using it all the time. You'd be wise to learn to think before you act. You are likely to be a cheerful, happy-go-lucky person but you need to be a bit more serious about things which matter.

If you answered mainly c) questions then you're either very short on common-sense or you haven't taken enough care with your replies. You could be a slightly anxious person who makes mistakes because you are easily flustered. Or you could be plain disinterested and believe that good health is a matter of pure luck. Whichever you are, take more care of yourself!

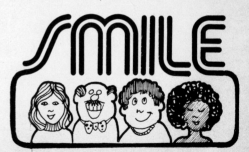

Dear Magazine

'I am very much in love with a girl and we plan to get married when I have finished my studies. But that won't be for another two years. And the waiting time is putting a great strain on our relationship. We quarrel a lot and it is usually my fault.

The trouble is that I want to make love to her. But she won't let me. She says she is afraid. She says we must wait till we're married. I tell her she is old-fashioned and that she doesn't love me enough. Please help me to change her mind.'

'My boyfriend and I have been living together for the past three months. This makes my Mum unhappy and my Dad won't have me in the house again. I love them both and don't want to hurt them. How can I make them see that it is my life and I have to make my own decisions?

My boyfriend and I are very happy but we've already found out that living together isn't always easy. What with his smelly socks; my hair curlers; never having enough money to do what we want! But I think all young people should have 'trial' marriages. Then there wouldn't be such a high divorce rate from early marriages.'

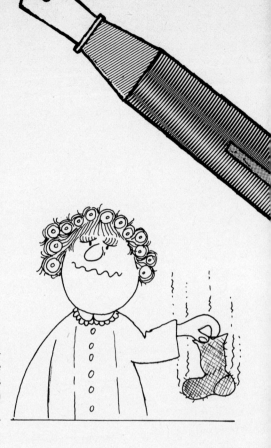

Many of our readers send us letters like these every week. They are not easy to answer. There are never any simple answers to human problems.

People are different. They are individuals with different standards, different needs, different dreams. What suits one person doesn't necessarily suit another. A great deal of harm can be done by trying to persuade someone to 'go against their feelings'. We need to respect the way another person thinks and feels. If we don't we risk great misery, both to the person we love and to ourselves. We can cause an awful lot of emotional damage if we are not very careful and very thoughtful.

Read these two letters again. You will notice how very different the problems are. There is a lot to discuss and think about in both situations.

Contraception

	TYPE	HOW SAFE	USED BY	METHOD
	THE PILL	Very safe	Woman	Follow instructions on packet
	THE SHEATH (condoms, Durex, rubbers, French letters)	Quite safe	Man	Put on before sexual intercourse (Use with spermicide)
	THE IUD (coil or loop)	Very safe	Woman	Put inside womb by a doctor
	THE DIAPHRAGM (Dutch cap)	Safe	Woman	Put at top of vagina before intercourse (Use with spermicide)
	SPERMICIDES (sperm killers – creams, jellies, foams)	Not very safe	Woman	Put inside vagina before intercourse
	THE 'SAFE' PERIOD (chart method)	Not safe	Both	10 days 'safe' in each month
	STERILISATION	Very safe	Man Woman	Vasectomy Sterilisation

BIRTH CONTROL

Whatever decisions people make they should know about birth control. There are serious reasons why. Unwanted babies – or babies born to unmarried mothers – often have an unhappy start in life. Young married couples need time to build a home together before they start their families. It is now known that babies born to *very* young parents may not be as happy or as healthy as babies born to older parents. We may feel we can take risks with our *own* future. But what about our children's future? (See 'Orphan Annie's' letter on page 7.)

Society is concerned about the damage done to unwanted children. We are all responsible to society for the health and happiness of our families. Birth Control and advice on what method to use is now free at the Family Planning Clinics. The Brook Advisory Centre for Young People is experienced in helping young unmarrieds with any birth control problem they may have. Do you think this picture 'works'? Have a discussion about it.

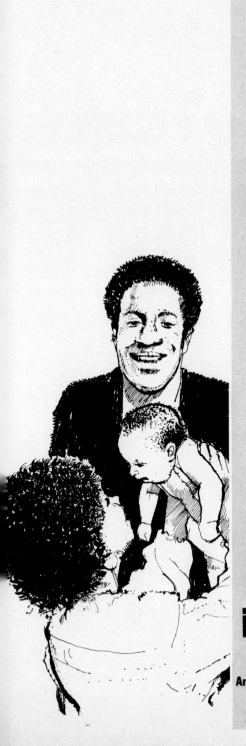

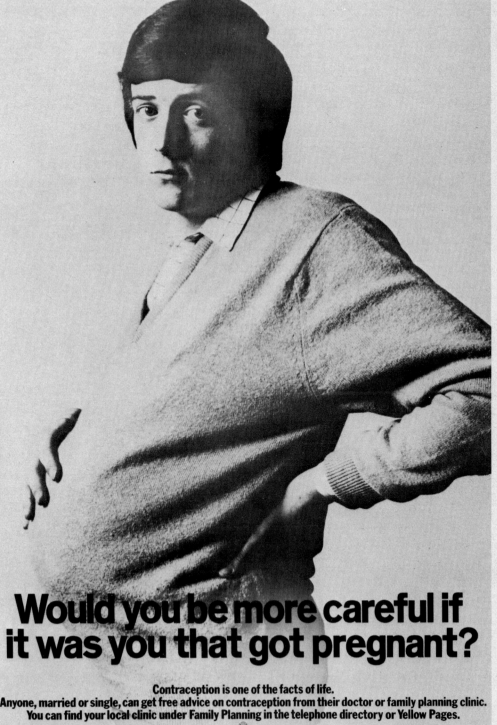

Would you be more careful if it was you that got pregnant?

Contraception is one of the facts of life.
Anyone, married or single, can get free advice on contraception from their doctor or family planning clinic.
You can find your local clinic under Family Planning in the telephone directory or Yellow Pages.

The Health Education Council
78 New Oxford Street, London WC1A 1AH.

Health People 2

The Midwife

I'm called a docimiliary midwife because I deliver babies at home. Nowadays most first babies are born in hospital. This means my mums have been through it all before.

It's not possible to describe a typical day. There's no such thing in my job. Babies have their own views on when they want to be born! So I'll tell you about Jenny Jones whose baby was born yesterday.

Her husband, Jim, rang at lunch time. He said her contractions had started. Contractions are caused by the powerful muscles of the womb beginning to push the baby down. I went straight round there. Jenny was sitting in her dressing gown playing with her little girl. Together we prepared the bedroom, clearing the dressing table and spreading out the pre-packed sterile equipment. I check the gowns, masks, gloves, caps, towels and syringes. I *always* bring an extra pack – to be on the safe side.

Jenny's neighbour drops in and this gives me the chance to return to the office. I leave a message stating where I am and collect the drugs and Trilene. Second babies often come quickly so I hurry back.

I examine Jenny internally. The cervix, a strong ring of muscles at the top of the vagina, is beginning to open. I judge it will take about another two hours. I listen to the baby's heart beat. Steady as a drum. Excellent. We go back into the sitting-room and have a cup of coffee. Jenny is tensing up against the contractions.

Her neighbour notices this. Suddenly she pretends *she* is having a contraction. We all laugh. I can see it makes Jenny more relaxed. I tell a few jokes about funny things that have happened during other deliveries. We giggle quite a bit. Jenny is now cheerful and calm. That's how I want it to be. None of this solemn stuff. Happy mums have much easier births.

Jim gets back from work and the neighbour takes the little girl home with her. We get Jenny onto the bed. She's having quite painful contractions now so I place the Trilene near her on the bedside table. It's a mixture of pain-killing gas and air in a handy container. She is going to try not to use it (it's better for the baby) but she feels safe knowing it is there. Jim strokes her hand when she moans.

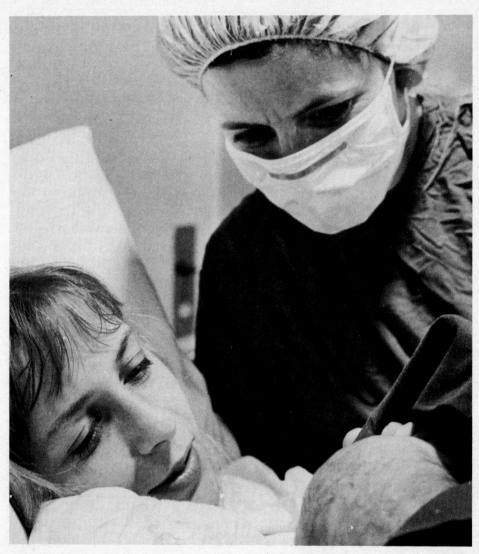

At last the cervix is fully dilated (opened). I send Jim out to scrub up and put on a sterile gown and mask. Jenny begins the second stage of labour. The waters break and she feels huge bearing-down pains. The baby's head can be seen and I concentrate totally on keeping the delivery steady; not too fast – not too slow.

Then Jim is beside me cheering and egging her on as if she were a footballer about to kick the winning goal! Jenny gives a loud cry as the head is born. She half sits up to watch as her baby son enters this world. It is a wonderful moment for all of us.

The baby takes a deep breath and lets out a yell of protest. That's the sound I like to hear. It tells me he is breathing strongly. Then I put clamps on the cord, suck through a special tube to make sure his lungs are clear and put drops in his eyes. Jim holds him close to Jenny.

The third stage of labour is the 'afterbirth'. This is made up of the placenta, the cord and the membranes protecting the baby. The afterbirth usually comes about ten minutes later. I check it to make sure it has all come away. Then I freshen Jenny up, do a detailed check of the baby's development and get them both ready for breast-feeding.

New borns aren't really hungry but they can suck for a short while. Jenny knows exactly how to hold him and they settle together comfortably. This early bit of breast-feeding brings mum and baby very close together. The sucking also helps Jenny's milk to start flowing. Jim helps me to clear up my equipment – then pops next door to bring back their little girl. As she is held up to meet her baby brother I close the door quietly and leave. The picture of this happy family will stay with me for a long while.

When I get back to the office I realise how exhausted I am. It's nearly midnight before I finish my paperwork. For a midwife, there is always some tension during the delivery. A slow birth means the baby may get short of oxygen. A painful birth means the administration of drugs which often affect the baby. The 'counting-of-toes', checking to make sure the baby is properly developed, is a bit tension-making too. It's terribly upsetting if something is found to be wrong.

But I love my work. It's rare for things to go wrong. If they do, I call the family doctor, the ambulance of the 'baby flying squad' depending on the extent of the emergency. But as Jenny had attended all the ante-natal sessions and was in perfect health I had a feeling this would be a safe and easy delivery.

Tomorrow and for the next two weeks I will visit daily. The family doctor will also do a more detailed examination of both mother and baby. After that Jenny will bring her baby to the Child Health Centre for checks on his progress, for vaccinations, for free milk coupons, vitamin tablets, advice on contraception or just a friendly chat. If for some reason she doesn't attend, the health visitor will go round to make sure everything is progressing well. We do our best to look after our babies!

Our midwife is employed by the National Health Service. Since 1974 the Social Service and the National Health Service have been combined to form the Department of Health and Social Security – the DHSS. The function of the DHSS is to care for the health and welfare of the community. A large part of this care is *preventive* medicine and aid. Preventive work is to *stop things going wrong* before or as they start. The early vaccination of infants and small children to protect them from diseases which were killers is one of the most successful forms of preventive medicine.

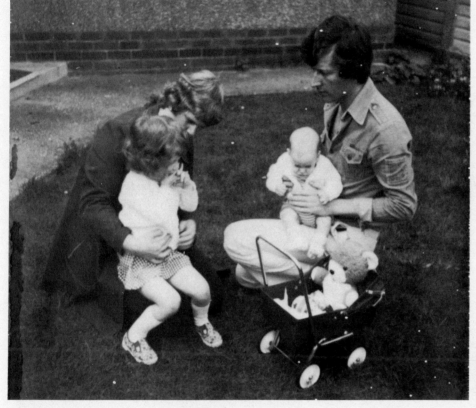

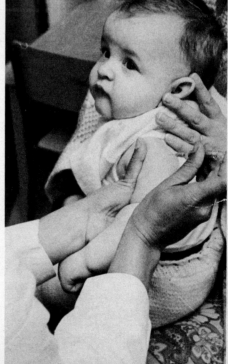

AGE	VACCINATION
4 to 6 months	Diptheria, tetanus and whooping cough given as one injection. Polio vaccine taken by mouth. Dose I.
6 to 8 weeks later	The same as above. Dose II.
11 to 13 months	The same as above. Dose III.
2 to 3 years	Measles vaccine.
5 years	Diphtheria and tetanus 'booster'. Polio 'booster'.
11 years	Rubella vaccine for girls against German measles.
10 to 13 years	B.C.G. against tuberculosis (T.B.).
15 years	Booster vaccine tetanus, polio. Maybe smallpox.

Find out about and discuss:
The importance of regular ante-natal visits.
Diet, exercise and health during pregnancy.
Fathers being present at the birth.
Hospital or Home? (Some mothers prefer to have their second baby at home.)
The work of the National Childbirth Trust.
The importance of regular visits to the Child Health Centre.

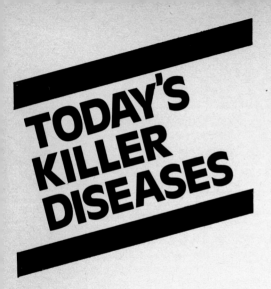

TODAY'S KILLER DISEASES

No wonder smokers cough.

The tar and discharge that collects in the lungs of an average smoker.

One hundred years ago the top killer diseases included typhoid, tuberculosis, diphtheria, scarlet fever, pneumonia and cholera. Since then improved housing, immunisation, clean water supplies, safe sewage disposal, better standards of nutrition and the discovery of new drugs e.g. antibiotics have wiped away most of these diseases.

Today's top killers include heart attacks, strokes, bronchitis, lung cancer, stomach ulcers, stomach cancers and accidents. While scientists are working on research against these diseases, we can take certain *preventive* action ourselves – to cut down on any unnecessary risks.

Heart attacks and strokes: Get enough exercise, diet if overweight, try to avoid emotional stress, reduce the amount of animal fats in diet, cut out smoking completely.

Bronchitis and Lung cancer: Take an active part in schemes to prevent air pollution (smokeless fuels, motor exhausts, factory fumes). Insist on the safety air regulations in dusty occupations. Stop self-pollution by refusing to smoke cigarettes.

Stomach ulcers and cancers: The causes of these are not fully known but stress and smoking are thought to aggravate stomach ulcers.

Accidents: In the 15 to 44 age group, fatal accidents (and suicides) account for 1 in 3 deaths amongst men; 1 in 6 deaths amongst women. Fatal accidents at work average about 2,000 each year; 7,000 people are killed on the roads; 8,000 are killed in their homes. Human error is responsible for nearly all accidents.

It has been estimated that for every person killed in an accident, there are ten others seriously injured for life. For the next thirty years you will be most at risk from an accident! So take care! However, if you are smoking during that time, you risk the other killer diseases in middle age.

* 66 British people die of bronchitis every day. Of these, no more than 3 will be non-smokers living in the country.
* Each time a cigarette is smoked 20 to 30 milligrams of vitamin C is used up.
* More people are regular users of tobacco than any other drug.
* 13 times more smokers than non-smokers die of lung cancer.
* Cigarette smoking is responsible for more deaths from bronchitis and lung cancer than all deaths due to accidents, infectious diseases, alcohol and stomach cancer put together.

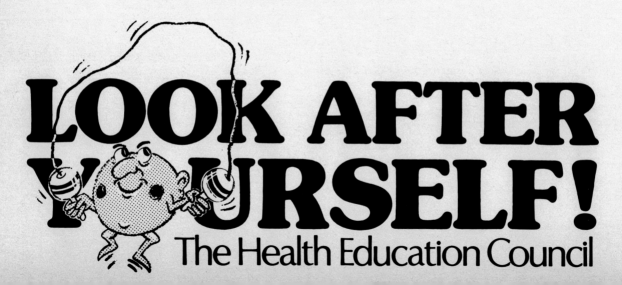

LOOK AFTER YOURSELF!
The Health Education Council

Dear Sally Wise

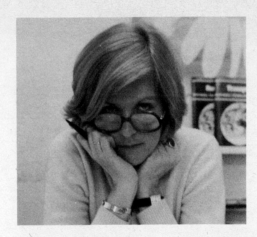

DEAR SALLY WISE,

My oldest sister is expecting her first baby and we are all excited about it. My problem is this. She is a heavy smoker – at least 20 cigarettes a day – and I'm afraid for the health of the baby inside her. I have told her to stop smoking but she only laughs at me. Her husband agrees with her and calls me a 'silly worrier'. What can I do? She reads this magazine and might take some notice of what you say.

It is always difficult to persuade people to stop doing what they want to do. Especially when they are 'hooked', as your sister and her husband obviously are. But you are right to be worried and to try to stop them.

It is a well-established fact that babies born to smoking mothers are not as healthy as other babies. It has also been found that by the age of 7 these children are shorter, don't read as well and are less well-adjusted than other children. These are harsh truths. They (and those about lung cancer, heart disease, etc.) are now being taught to all schoolchildren.

It is especially important for girls to understand that *if they begin smoking*, they may be hurting two people in the future. During the five to seven minutes it takes to smoke a cigarette the unborn baby has his oxygen supply cut short. A good and steady supply of oxygen is essential for the baby's development, especially of his heart, lungs and brain cells. At the same time as he is short of oxygen, he receives a damaging mixture of nicotine and other chemicals and gases in tobacco smoke. They pass directly to him from his mother's blood. As your sister is smoking 20 cigarettes a day, this happens to him 20 times a day.

If your sister needs any more convincing, tell her that most doctors – once the heaviest group of smokers – have given up the 'filthy weed'. Some hospitals refuse treatment to a patient who continues smoking. Your sister's

husband should also stop smoking. Otherwise she will go on breathing in the smoke from his cigarettes. Cigarette smokers pollute the air for those around them.

Keep plugging away at your sister and her husband. That beautiful baby will have an aunt he or she can be really proud of!

Write to ASH (Action on Smoking and Health) and the Health Education Council for more information on the dangers of smoking. (Always send a stamped addressed envelope.) Work out a project for teaching 8 and 9-year-olds why they should not begin smoking.

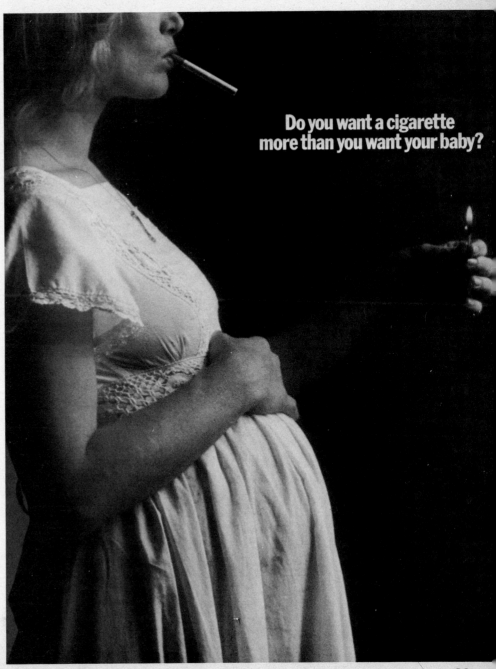

Do you want a cigarette more than you want your baby?

DEAR SALLY WISE,

Mark and me (I'm Gary) have some fairly wild friends. We went to a party they threw in their new flat last week. Everyone seemed to be tripping. They tried to persuade us to take some acid but we didn't want to. So they threw us out! We don't want to lose them as friends. What should we do?

Nothing, I'm afraid. From a purely practical point of view you would be wise not to visit them again. They could be raided at any time by the police who usually know where drug parties are held. You could be arrested as well. It is always sad to lose friends but drug-takers are immature people who want to escape from their problems. It seems to me that you and Mark have outgrown 'wild friends', as you call them.

Write to the Information Officer of the Institute for the Study of Drug Dependence for suggestions for books, films, wallcharts and other material suitable for further study.

DEAR SALLY WISE,

I must have very sensitive ears or something. I absolutely cannot stand the noise at discos. Nor can I bear the radio or telly turned up full blast. It sets off a throbbing deep inside my head. And then I get unbearable headaches. But I seem such a spoil-sport if I ask for the sound to be turned down.

Poor you. You are one of the many people who suffer from *noise pollution*. Amplified pop music has risen to third place in the noise league table. It is now regarded as a serious health hazard as it can lead to loss of hearing.

Loud persistent noise damages in two ways. The tiny hair cells in the inner ear which pick up the sound vibrations become worn away. We lose our hearing. This is physical damage. But relentless loud noise also causes mental damage. We become irritable, then angry. Noise can be infuriating and many accidents are caused from its effect on us.

I'm afraid there isn't much you can do except keep well clear of noisy places. Find a companion who likes walks in the country. Find a hobby which is interesting *and* social but quiet. Insist that the noise is turned down in your home. (If you must go to discos wear wax plugs in your ears.)

Find out about other forms of noise pollution by writing to the Noise Abatement Society. 'There has to be a reason why the kids of today play their music so loudly.' Can you think of any reasons? Think carefully before you discuss this.

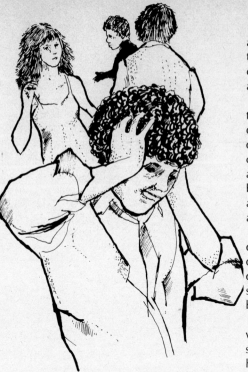

To Miss Northumbria: My advice is to drop him immediately. A boy who strikes his girl during the courting stage is quite likely to become brutally violent after marriage. Do it now. Don't wait for another boy to come along as a replacement. That would be unfair and provoke attacks of the violent jealousy which you are so frightened of. Don't think you can change this boy. You can't. Take your courage in your hands and gently break it off for good.

When courting, people are usually on their best behaviour. Miss Northumbria's fiance is already behaving brutally to her. It is important she knows that people *do not change* just because they get married. This is true of most vicious or bad behaviour. If she goes ahead with the wedding plans she may well end up as a battered wife.

DEAR SALLY WISE,

I have an extraordinary girlfriend. Her boast is she can drink any one of us – me and my mates – under the table. And she can ! The one time I took on her challenge I ended up vomiting horribly in the street and feeling as if I was going to die. She just jeered at me and went off with another bloke. What I want to know is how can she drink so much when 4 pints make me so ill?

Well, yes, your girlfriend does sound extraordinary. But she also sounds as if she isn't very fond of you. Have you thought of that?

To answer your question: alcohol is an *addictive* drug. People who drink heavily build up a *tolerance* to the poisons in alcohol. Gradually the cells of the body get to need larger and larger doses. The person craves alcohol. They are addicted. It requires a great deal of alcohol to satisfy the cravings.

You are not an alcoholic so your stomach throws out the excess alcohol when you drink 4 pints. However, if you continued to drink this much each evening, *your* body cells would also develop a tolerance to alcohol. You could 'hold' far more drink before being sick or passing out. You would also be well on the way to becoming an alcoholic.

Alcohol is the most commonly abused drug. It is also one of the most dangerous drugs in our society. Any form of heavy drinking is a tragic problem. Slowly but steadily the whole personality of the drinker begins to break up and disintegrate.

Your girlfriend sounds seriously ill – as well as being mentally unwell. Try to persuade her to get help from a doctor. Take her to the organisation, Alcoholics Anonymous. Alcoholism can be cured but it is a long, difficult and painful road. Your girlfriend will need courage and friendship to see her through.

Whatever you decide to do about your relationship with this girl – don't try to keep up with her drinking. That would simply be disaster for both of you.

Find out about the work of the AA (Alcoholics Anonymous) and of the National Council on Alcoholism. Heavy drinking is becoming a serious and sad problem amongst young people. It is one of the most dangerous health hazards. You need to know as much as possible about this subject.

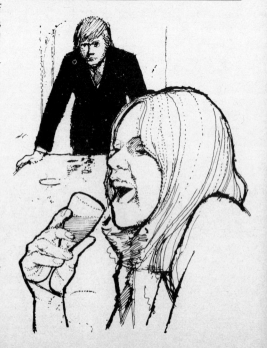

they call me FOUR EYES

I started wearing glasses when I first went to school. The teacher noticed I couldn't see what was written on the blackboard too clearly.

She brought me up to the front of the class and she told mum. I was taken to the optician and fitted with National Health specs. Mum gulped when she first saw me wearing them. 'Poor little boy', she kept saying, which irritated me.

I've worn glasses ever since and I've got used to being called 'four-eyes' now. It's one of those boring things other people always say. They think it's witty. I just crack my face in a polite smile. But I wish they wouldn't think they've said something clever. It's so corny. I've heard it a million times. As I say, it's just something you have to put up with.

But what I don't understand is why I'm taken for a serious sort of person. Just because I wear glasses. I've got a lazy mind and I don't care who knows it. A glance at the newspaper and checking my pools coupons is the nearest I get to studying. But as soon as people see my glasses they think 'Oh, there's a brainy bloke.' Daft!

I've just got the wrong size eyeballs. (I was born with them and I'll die with them.) It sounds funny, I know, but it's true. They are too long, my eyeballs. When distant light rays come into my eye, they don't land in a

neat point at the back. Because my eye is too long. The rays spread and I get a blurred image. So I wear extra lenses – which is all glasses really are – to bend the distant light rays so they land all together on the retina. That's the place at the back of the eye where you get a nice, sharp picture.

Being short-sighted isn't too bad. If I don't wear my specs I have to be careful not to bump into street lamps and then apologise

to them thinking I've knocked into a pedestrian. And the other thing is when you fancy the look of a girl at a disco. By the time you've gone over to her and asked her to dance, you're stuck with her. I can't get a really good look until I'm up close!

But now a real crisis has arisen at home. My sister Sue, who is 16, has been told she is short-sighted too, though not as badly as I am. She's throwing hysterics. She's abso-

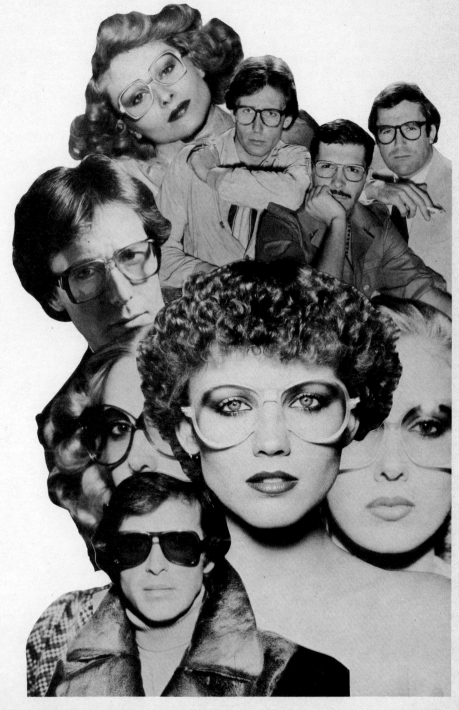

lutely refusing to wear glasses.

'It's all right for him,' she says pointing at me. 'Men don't look too bad in glasses. They look kind of steady and decent and reliable. And anyway, girls aren't put off by men wearing glasses.' Then she adds very angry, 'Didn't you know the saying – "Men never make passes at girls who wear glasses".' Poor kid.

I wonder if that saying is true? I wouldn't know because I'm so used to wearing them I hardly notice them on a girl. I do hope it isn't true. What with all this Women's Lib around – and the way they are making us feel chauvinistic pigs – it would be one more weapon they could throw at us.

Anyway, there is Sue at home screaming a lot of rubbish about losing her good looks. Mum is terrified Sue'll be attacked by rapists because she won't be able to see them coming, would you believe? Even Dad is joining in, though with more sense. He's worried Sue will get herself run over if she can't see the traffic. And both Mum and Dad are turning on *me* to try to persuade Sue to wear her glasses.

As you can imagine, Sue won't listen to anything *I* say about it. What a scene. Help!

CONTACT LENSES

Sue could try wearing contact lenses. They are very small and fit over the iris and pupil. She will need to be shown how to slip them on to the front of her eyes. At first they may feel bulky, they may cause a little irritation. But as she gets used to them she will almost forget she is wearing them. A few people cannot bear the idea of putting anything onto their eyes and they never manage to wear contact lenses. However Sue does sound very determined *not* to wear glasses. She may have great success with contact lenses.

Contact lenses are expensive to make and to buy. They are usually not given free on the National Health Service. It is wise to have them insured as they are so small and transparent they are often dropped and can't be found again. It is also sensible to keep your glasses for wearing at home, or when your eyes are tired, or in case of any eye infection.

EYE-CARE

Behind the pupil of the eye is a lens. This is pulled forward till it becomes thicker when we do close work. It is pulled thinner for when we look at distant objects. The muscles which pull on the lens may become very tired when we do a lot of close study. Students should stare off into the distance – out of the window at chimneys and so on – for a few minutes to rest these muscles during long periods of study.

Daylight or artificial light should fall directly onto the work we are doing. This causes the least strain on our eyes.

Always wear a helmet with visor when on a motorbike.

Wear protective, shatter-proof goggles when doing dangerous work.

The most common eye infection is conjunctivitis or 'pink eye'. It is caused by tiny germs from dirty towels, face cloths, hankies or grubby hands. It is very infectious and should be treated as soon as possible.

By middle age most people find small print difficult and need glasses for reading.

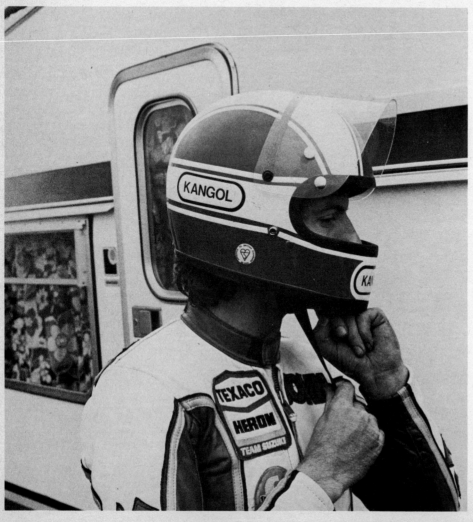

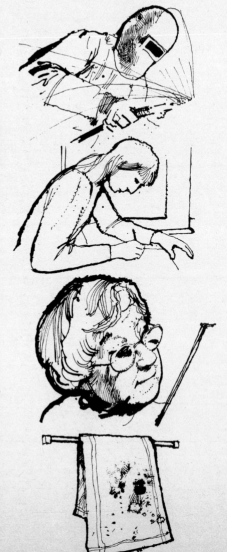

MONEY MATTERS

The D.H.S.S. – the National Health Service and the Social Security Services are huge organisations and very very expensive to run. The money to finance the D.H.S.S. is collected from us in two main ways.

1. National Insurance Contributions which every working person must pay.
2. The Consolidated Fund which is a complicated source of money collected directly and indirectly from us in different taxes.

National Insurance contributions are paid partly by the employer and partly by the employee. Both contributions are usually paid as the wage packets are made up. Your contribution will be taken from your wages before you receive them. If you are self-employed you are bound by law to make sure you pay your full contribution.

The Consolidated Fund from taxes and the National Insurance contributions act as joint insurances to cover you in times of financial difficulties, ill-health and old age.

These include Maternity Benefits and Grants, Child Benefit, Sickness Benefit, Unemployment and Pension Rights.

There are many areas in which state insurance also helps, e.g.:

A *Mobility Allowance* for physically handicapped people.

An *Invalid Allowance* and *Pension* if you are still unfit to work after 28 weeks illness.

An *Invalid Care Allowance* for people who could work but stay at home to care for a severely disabled relative.

An *Attendance Allowance* for severely disabled people who need a lot of looking after. The benefit is higher for people who need attendance by day *and* by night.

A *Death Grant* to help cover the expenses of a funeral.

SUPPLEMENTARY BENEFITS

These are cash benefits paid if you are *not* in full-time work and your income (if any) is too low to live on. You do not have to have paid any contributions. Benefit is paid as a *right* providing you satisfy the social security office of your low income and your needs.

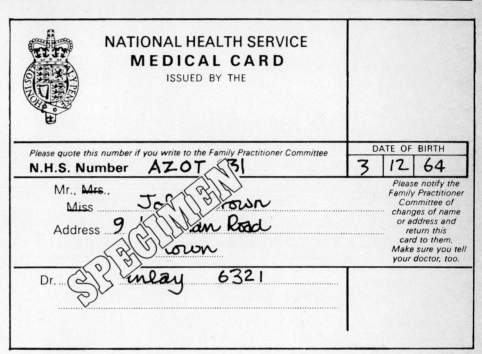

| | | DATE OF BIRTH |
NATIONAL HEALTH SERVICE **MEDICAL CARD** ISSUED BY THE

Please quote this number if you write to the Family Practitioner Committee

N.H.S. Number   AZOT 31

DATE OF BIRTH   3 12 64

Mr., Mrs., Miss

Address

Dr.

Please notify the Family Practitioner Committee of changes of name or address and return this card to them. Make sure you tell your doctor, too.

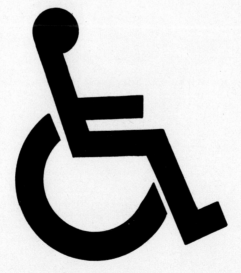

SUPPLEMENTARY PENSIONS

These are paid to people over retirement age who are not in full-time work.

SUPPLEMENTARY ALLOWANCES

These are additional benefits which can be paid to people in full-time work but whose income is below a certain level. These other benefits you can get include:

Free prescriptions.

Free milk and vitamins for expectant mothers and children under school age.

Free dental treatment, false teeth and glasses.

Free school meals.

Hospital fares for patients who have to visit hospital regularly.

Legal aid and advice.

Rent and rate rebates and rent allowances.

There are many ways in which people in need can be helped. As money becomes available or as different needs arise benefits are changed. Always ask your social security officer for all the ways in which you can be helped.

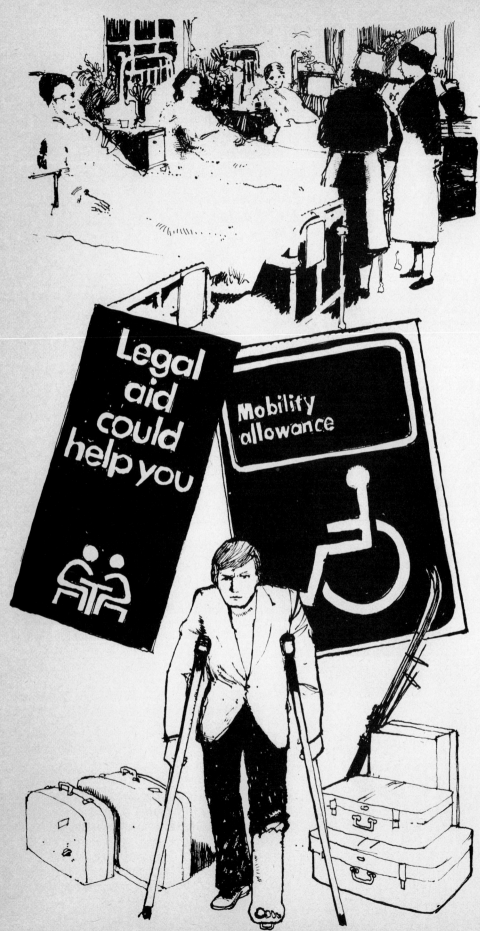

SICKNESS BENEFIT

You are entitled to free medical care once you have signed on with a doctor and received your medical health card. When you are unable to go to work through illness, you are entitled to claim sickness benefit. But it is you who has to make the claim. Your employer will not do it for you.

Once you have had your illness diagnosed, your doctor will tell you how long you are likely to be off sick. Before you leave the surgery, make sure you have the claim form for sickness benefit. Sign it and post it to your local social security office as *soon as possible*. Otherwise you may lose the benefit for that particular week. If you are too ill to get to the post-box you must find a friend to do it for you.

You will also need a doctor's certificate to claim for the invalid benefits.

TEMPORARY ABSENCE FROM HOME

You are entitled to free medical care wherever you stay in the United Kingdom. If you get sick while on holiday or if your work involves travelling across the country, apply to the nearest doctor as a temporary resident. Give your National Health Service Number and the name and address of your own doctor. You may be a temporary resident for up to 3 months. If you stay away from home for more than 3 months after you sign on, you should register with the new doctor. Children at boarding school and students at college or university are usually on the register with a doctor in the place where they are studying.

TEMPORARY ABSENCE ABROAD

The cost of medical treatment is very expensive. British citizens are entitled to free treatment when they visit any of the EEC countries. You are entitled to the same standard of treatment as the citizens of these countries receive. You may not demand any extra treatment unless you are prepared to pay for it. You *must* carry the form E111 with you and show it to the medical authorities. You can get this form from any health or social security office before you leave.

If you are travelling outside an EEC country it is wise to take out a private health insurance. It doesn't cost much. But treatment for a broken leg, an infected finger, food poisoning or any illness could cost you your next year's earnings. A private health insurance isn't exactly preventive medicine – it's more like preventive financial disaster!

useful addresses

Age Concern, see local telephone directory for your nearest branch.

Alcoholics Anonymous, see local telephone directory. Head office, 11 Redcliffe Gardens, London SW10 9BG.

Action on Smoking and Health Ltd (ASH), 27 Mortimer Street, London W1N 7RJ.

British Pregnancy Advisory Service, see local telephone directory.

Brook Advisory Centres, Central Office, 233 Tottenham Court Road, London W1P 9AE. For information on contraception.

Christian Aid, Headquarters, 2 Sloane Gardens, London SW1W 9BW.

Citizens Advice Bureau, see local telephone directory.

Community Services Volunteers, 237 Pentonville Road, London N1 9NG.

Contact (Helping the Elderly), 15 Henrietta Street, London WC2E 8QH. Welcomes volunteers with cars.

Dr. Barnardo's, Head Office, Tanners Lane, Barkingside, Ilford 1G6 1QG, Essex.

Family Planning Association, National Office, 27 Mortimer Street, London W1N 7RJ.

General Dental Council, 37 Wimpole Street, London W1M 7AE.

Health Education Council, 78 New Oxford Street, London WC1A 1HB.

Health Education Office, see local telephone directory.

Help the Aged, Head Office, 8 Denman Street, London W1V 7RF; Education Department, 157 Waterloo Road, London SE1 8XN.

Institute for the Study of Drug Dependence, 3 Blackburn Road, London NW6 1RZ.

International Voluntary Service, Head Office, 53 Regent Road, Leicester LE1 6YL.

Invalid Children's Aid Association, Central Office, 126 Buckingham Palace Road, London SW1W 9SA.

Liberation Films, 2 Chichele Road, London NW2 3DA; excellent short 'Trigger' films to stimulate discussion on emotional, social and health topics.

London Youth Advisory Centre, 26 Prince of Wales Road, Kentish Town, London NW5 3LG.

National Association for Mental Health (MIND), Harmont House, 22 Harley Street, London W1N 2ED.

National Blood Transfusion Service, see local telephone directory.

National Childbirth Trust, 9 Queensborough Terrace, London W2 3TB.

National Children's Bureau, 8 Wakly Street, London EC1V 7QE.

National Council on Alcoholism, 3 Grosvenor Crescent, London SW1X 7EE.

National Society for the Prevention of Cruelty to Children (NSPCC), National Headquarters, 1 Riding House Street, London W1P 7PA.

Noise Abatement Society, 6 Old Bond Street, London W1X 3TA.

Oxfam, Head Office, 274 Banbury Road, Oxford OX2 7DZ.

Physical Education Association of Great Britain and Northern Ireland, 10 Nottingham Place, London W1M 3FA. For information on interesting and unusual sports and activities.

Physically Handicapped and Able-Bodied (PHAB), 42 Devonshire Street, London W1N 1LN.

Pre-School Playgroups Association (PPA), Headquarters, Alford House, Aveline Street, London SE11 5DH.

Release, 1 Elgin Avenue, London W9 3PR. Gives advice to young people in trouble over drug dependence.

Royal Society for the Prevention of Accidents (RoSPA), 1 Grosvenor Crescent, London SW1X 7EE.

Save the Children Fund, Head Office, 157 Clapham Road, London SW9 0PU.

Task Force, Headquarters, Clifford House, Edith Villas, London W14 8UG.

War on Want. Head Office, 467 Caledonian Road, London, N7 9BA.

Young Volunteer Force Foundation, 7 Leonard Street, London EC2A 4AQ.

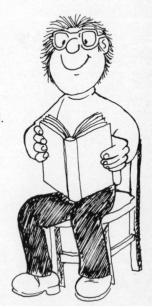